52
WAYS TO
LOSE
WEIGHT

52 WAYS TO LOSE WEIGHT

Carl Dreizler
and
Mary E. Ehemann

A Division of Thomas Nelson Publishers
Nashville

To our coworkers
at New Life Treatment Centers
and to the many lives
we've seen changed here

Carl and Mary

And especially
to my best friend Sharon
who has faithfully walked with me
to reach freedom in Him

Mary

Copyright © 1992 by Stephen Arterburn, Carl Dreizler, and Mary E.
Ehemann

Published in Nashville, Tennessee, by Oliver-Nelson Books, a division of
Thomas Nelson, Inc., Publishers, and distributed in Canada by Lawson
Falle, Ltd., Cambridge, Ontario.

Unless otherwise noted, the Bible version used in this publication is THE
NEW KING JAMES VERSION. Copyright © 1979, 1980, 1982, Thomas
Nelson, Inc., Publishers.

Printed in the United States of America.

Library of Congress Cataloging-in-Publication Data

Dreizler, Carl, 1954–
    52 ways to lose weight / Carl Dreizler & Mary E. Ehemann.
        p.   cm.
    ISBN 0-8407-9605-6 (pbk.)
    1. Reducing.   I. Ehemann, Mary E., 1955–   . II. Title.   III. Title:
Fifty-two ways to lose weight.
RM222.2.D7   1992
613.2′5—dc20   91-33640
                                                                 CIP

1 2 3 4 5 6 — 97 96 95 94 93 92

Contents

Introduction

Whether you are reading this book to lose 20 or 120 pounds, you will find most of the fifty-two ways are small steps that lead to big success in your quest to be slimmer and healthier.

In the pages that follow we do not present one short-term fad diet after another. Fad diets often are used to lose a certain amount of weight. Yet once the diet is terminated, the weight creeps back. Instead, we hope you will use the ideas to completely change the way you eat *and think* for the rest of your life.

The problem of excess weight is not strictly physical in most cases. Much of the problem centers on the need to create new behavioral patterns and a healthier self-image. Therefore, the chapters in this book focus on three primary perspectives: physical, emotional, and spiritual.

- **Physical.** Practical suggestions are provided for replacing higher-calorie foods with lower-calorie foods. Fats, cholesterol, and other components that contribute to weight gain will be considered. Many actual recipes are included.

Instructional chapters will teach you to eat fewer foods containing sodium and to count daily calorie intake more carefully. Several different ideas are given for setting up regular exercise as an essential part of your weight-loss routine.

- **Emotional.** Many practical chapters help you to assess your current eating patterns, encourage you to chart your daily intake of food, and help you to come face to face with some of the issues that might be causing you to overeat. If you have gone from diet to diet only to get frustrated when the weight loss is only minimal or temporary, perhaps you have never concentrated on the parts of your life that might be causing you to consider food a loyal friend rather than a means of nutritional support. The principles contained herein will bring you to a new understanding and love for yourself.

- **Spiritual.** As human beings, we can do very little alone. We need the encouragement and support of friends. But even more, when the walls of our self-image have collapsed, we cannot rebuild them without the help of someone who loves us just as we are! For the two of us, that someone is Jesus Christ. Some of the following chapters focus upon this source of encouragement during your weight-loss program.

We sincerely believe that eating the right foods alone will not help the majority of people who are overweight. Rather, a transformation must take place within those people who want to become healthier. Real change can only take place if there is physical, emotional, and spiritual renewal. Since this is not a medical book, we recommend that anyone interested in losing a great deal of weight should consult a doctor. Our hope is that your life will be changed, if only by fewer pounds and a brighter, happier you!

1 TESTING ONE, TWO, THREE

Whether you are trying to lose those few inches that have mysteriously crept out from your body nearly hiding your view of your feet or whether you are battling a major weight problem, it is important that you do some self-analysis to determine how serious your eating problems have become.

The Principle You may need to begin eating healthier meals and to change some bad habits you've built up over time. Or you may need to deal with compulsive eating. This is not a medical book designed to provide a prescription, however. You should see your physician for specific health and weight problems.

To help assess your eating habits, take the following test.

The Action To determine if you are a compulsive eater, answer yes or no to the following questions.

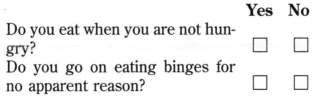

	Yes	No
1. Do you eat when you are not hungry?	☐	☐
2. Do you go on eating binges for no apparent reason?	☐	☐

	Yes	No
3. Do you have feelings of guilt or remorse after eating?	☐	☐
4. Do you give too much time and thought to food?	☐	☐
5. Do you look forward with pleasure and anticipation to moments of eating alone?	☐	☐
6. Do you plan secret binges ahead of time?	☐	☐
7. Do you eat sensibly with others but not when alone?	☐	☐
8. Is your weight affecting the way you live your life?	☐	☐
9. Have you tried to diet for a week (or longer) only to fall short of your goal?	☐	☐
10. Do you resent the advice of others who tell you to "use a little willpower" to stop overeating?	☐	☐
11. Despite evidence to the contrary, have you continued to boast that you can diet on your own whenever you wish?	☐	☐
12. Do you crave food at definite times of day or night other than mealtimes?	☐	☐
13. Do you eat to escape from worries or troubles?	☐	☐
14. Has your physician ever treated you for being overweight?	☐	☐

	Yes	**No**
15. Does your food obsession make you unhappy?	☐	☐

If you checked yes to three or more questions, you can benefit from this book and the education that is provided herein with regard to compulsive overeating.

- Compulsive overeaters suffer from a hidden disease that is chronic and progressive.
- Overeating affects the self-esteem of its victims. It ravages a person inside while others may be unaware of what is happening.
- Children who grow up in families where one or both parents are alcoholics are especially prone to developing compulsive overeating behavior.
- Obesity has usually been viewed as a self-control issue rather than an illness.

A hot air balloon must drop its sandbags before it can reach new highs. Your self-esteem can reach new levels if you commit to dropping the baggage from your past and moving forward toward recovery and weight loss.

2 COUNTING CALORIES

Unfortunately, you can't see the number of calories in certain foods just by looking at them. However, the result of eating high-calorie foods becomes quite visible on your body!

The Principle Many people don't even notice the fact that they are consuming foods with an excessive number of calories. That is, they don't notice it until the results show up around their hips, thighs and waistline. Even though you can't see calories, they are very real.

Food supplies energy to our bodies. And calories measure how much energy each type of food provides. Foods high in calories supply much more energy and foods that are low in calories supply very little. Our bodies need energy whether we are sitting, standing or sleeping, but we particularly need energy when we're physically active.

The Action Many of the calories we take in are burned off through things like running, swimming or playing tennis. Any calories that are not used up through exercise or other activities are converted by our bodies into fat. If your diet supplies more calories than your body uses, you will store the excess calories in this way.

- On the average, one pound of fat equals 3,500 calories. If you add 3,500 calories to the number of calories your body requires for normal energy requirements, you can gain a pound. But if you subtract 3,500 calories from your energy requirements, you can lose a pound.

- Applesauce has about 115 calories per portion because of the sugar content. Unsweetened applesauce contains only 50 calories per serving. The difference may not seem like much, but a savings of 65 calories each day for one year can mean a savings of almost 24,000 calories. This translates into seven fewer pounds resting uncomfortably around your midsection and other places.

- One medium avocado contains 425 calories, and yet avocados are considered a health food item. Adding some foods like avocados to your low-calorie salad may defeat your purpose.

We check the gas gauge and balance our checkbooks regularly. In much the same way, we need to track, document, and balance the amount and types of foods we eat.

3 I'M POSITIVE

One of the most vivid childhood stories that we can apply to our adult lives is the one about "The Little Train that Could." Turn your negative thoughts into "I think I can, I think I can, I think I can."

The Principle One of the reasons people don't lose weight is the fact that they make excuses. "Why should I go on a diet? I've never lost weight on one before." "I figure I'm so overweight already. What's one more piece of cake?" "I would exercise, but it only makes me tired and sore."

Part of your journey to lose weight should include a complete way of rethinking. Turn your negative, self-defeating talk into positive, self-affirming, and self-motivating talk.

The Action Every time you catch yourself caught in a cycle of negative talk, find a way to turn it into a positive. Then post the positive thought where you can easily see it. Here are some examples:

Negative Thought	Positive Thought
I can never stay on a diet. I have no willpower.	**I am not going on a "diet." I am learning new ways to eat the right foods so that I will look better, feel better and be happier.**

I don't want to exercise because I hate it and it's a waste of my time.	**I am making a choice to exercise because I want more energy. In fact, the more I exercise, the more I enjoy it.**
I've failed so I'm just going to give up.	**Mistakes provide opportunities to grow and learn. I'm going to start over and pick up where I was yesterday.**
I'll never lose the weight I want. It's hopeless.	**This time I am setting realistic goals and will take one day at a time.**

Write some of the negative things you say to yourself and then list your own positive responses. Practice them every day.

4 TABLE, PLEASE

Famous last words: "Since we're going out for a special dinner tonight, I'll put my diet on hold—just this once."

The Principle   If you are part of today's active lifestyle you probably go out to eat quite often. Perhaps your job is such that you often eat with clients or you travel so much that you eat almost every meal in a restaurant. When we get away from the discipline of our homes, we tend to allow ourselves to stray from the eating plan we have established. Restaurant eating is a special challenge for those who are trying to lose weight. But with proper planning, you can eat out regularly and lose weight.

The Action   Each time you enter a restaurant for a meal, set a goal to order only healthy items. You can have a great time and still enjoy a delicious meal. Here are some pointers to keep in mind when you dine out.

- Select your restaurant wisely. Many restaurants feature healthy menu choices.
- Scan the menu quickly to avoid temptation. Look especially at the section of the menu that features healthy and low-calorie choices.

- Order your food first so you won't be influenced by the choices of others.
- Ask the server to have your food prepared with as little fat as possible.
- Talk to friends during meals to get your mind off food. Avoid emotional conversations.
- Avoid ordering alcohol. Order mineral water with a slice of lemon.

5 THREE MEALS A DAY

Did you know that just 300 calories worth of snacking a day will add up to an additional 110,000 calories over a year's time? That's a lot of extra weight for a harmless little snack.

The Principle   Even if you eat three balanced and healthy meals a day, your between-meal snacking may be adding inches to your body.

A nutritional program aired on television said that Americans are suffering from serious health problems associated with eating high carbohydrate snacks between meals. Many snack items are also filled with sodium, which causes us to retain unwanted water.

The Action   You may have to change your current diet very little if you commit to cutting out all snacks and food between regular meals. If you give up snacking, you will likely learn to enjoy your meals more, and your body will have to work less to digest food with complex carbohydrates.

After you have made the adjustment to deleting all snacks from your diet, begin concentrating on eating healthier and lower-calorie meals for breakfast, lunch, and dinner. This will help you to drop even more inches and pounds. This gradual approach of first giving up snacking and then improving your diet may be an easier adjustment than simply going on a crash diet to change all your eating patterns. While the latter works well in theory, few people are able to stay with a program that introduces too many changes at once.

6 VEGETABLE SUBSTITUTES

If you were like most kids, you found ways to get rid of the vegetables from your dinner plate. Perhaps you used the hide-them-in-the-napkin trick or you hid them in the last inch of milk left in your glass. Here is a way for us to make vegetables our friends.

The Principle You can greatly reduce the calorie content of many recipes by replacing high-calorie ingredients with vegetables. Many people dislike the taste of vegetables, especially those loaded with vitamins. Vegetables such as broccoli, spinach, greens, and carrots may overpower sensitive taste buds if they are served alone.

The Action Adding vegetables to casseroles, sauces, dips, and soups will dilute their taste, yet add more flavor to the foods you are serving. Here are some suggestions for sneaking vegetables into your recipes:

- Grate or chop carrots and add them to your spaghetti sauce instead of meat. Cooked, chopped carrots have approximately the same texture as ground beef. Add mushrooms, zucchini, and onions to create a great vegetarian sauce greatly reduced in fat.
- For lasagne use chopped broccoli, spinach, or greens mixed with low-fat cottage cheese, noodles, and tomato sauce instead of beef.

- Mix chopped vegetables such as broccoli, greens, spinach, carrots, or squash with plain nonfat yogurt to create a delicious nonfat, vitamin-rich dip.
- To macaroni and cheese add broccoli, carrots, and cauliflower. Be sure to use a low-fat cheese and nonfat milk instead of cream in your recipe. You may want to try using fresh spinach pasta.
- If you want some meat in your diet, instead of standard meat loaf prepare vegetable beef loaf. Mix chopped cooked carrots and whole kernel corn with the leanest meat you can buy. Then add fresh herbs and spices.

We recommend that you find creative ways to make substitutions similar to the ones listed above in your favorite recipes. It is important when selecting your vegetables that you combine those that cook in relatively the same amount of time. For example, when combining carrots and broccoli, make sure the carrots are cooked first because they take longer to cook than does broccoli.

7 JOG YOUR MEMORY

There was a big woman in red
Who ate every bite she was fed
She wanted some changes
So now she arranges
To run off her largeness instead

The Principle An aerobic exercise that can contribute to your weight loss is regular jogging. If your memories of jogging bring back thoughts of boring trips around a track in high school or grueling pain and soreness afterward, you should give this exercise another try. There are things you can do to make jogging more fun and less painful. With modern technology you can wear headphones and listen to your favorite relaxing music, or use the time to converse with yourself or God regarding the changes you are making within yourself.

The Action Before you begin this or any other regular exercise, consult your physician. If you are extremely overweight, jogging can be stressful to your ankles, hips, and knees. If you have bursitis, back problems, or arthritis, jogging may not be for you.

Jogging will give you faster results than will walking. But if you have not exercised in a long time, consider a regular brisk walk for the first couple of weeks until you begin to get in shape. Begin your jogging with a short run for the next couple of weeks. Each week, increase the distance you run until you reach a predetermined goal, and stay with that distance for your regular exercise. Find out from a fitness expert what the ideal pulse rate is for a person of your age and weight before and after exercise. Use this measure as a guideline to your exertion level. Don't overdo it.

- Before jogging or any aerobic exercise, always do a set of stretching exercises that focus especially on your back, hamstrings, calves, and Achilles tendons.
- When picking your running terrain, try to find a level surface when you first begin. Running on hills can cause your body harm and should be attempted only by experienced joggers.
- Find a place that will make you feel good about being outside. Rather than running around the track at the local high school, find an open field, lakeshore, or seashore that has a safe path for your exercise.

Many people prefer to jog alone, however, you may want to find a friend to jog with you. This will help keep you committed to the schedule and will make the time more enjoyable.

8 STEP BY STEP

Running up and down the steps at the local high school stadium will probably work off some calories, but we recommend another set of steps too!

The Principle Some changes can take place fast. For example, you can change the color of your living room in just one day. Only a couple of steps are involved in this process: buy the paint and brush it on. But other changes, such as altering a habit that has been practiced for years, can only take place by following a more lengthy set of steps.

The Action A number of support groups offered through various organizations have sprung up in almost every part of the United States. Look in your telephone directory, ask your personal physician, or call your local Chamber of Commerce or church to locate a group that would be compatible with your needs.

Here are some general steps you need to take in order to take full advantage of these groups:

- Seek an assessment or diagnostic analysis from a qualified therapist, counselor, or doctor
- Call or write the group (using the above resources) for literature regarding the group's philosophy

- Locate a support group near you
- Commit yourself to attending as often as the group recommends
- Attend the group for the first time as an observer (see chapter 9)
- Make a commitment to become a regular participant in the group
- Be accountable for the assignments you are given
- Commit to staying with the group throughout your entire recovery process

You won't be responsible for losing pounds or, for that matter, completely changing your life overnight. You have the rest of your life to work on your recovery.

9 MORAL SUPPORT

Few of us have the ability to do everything on our own. When we are faced with a long journey we often need friends there to push us or carry us when the road gets weary.

The Principle Sometimes when we want to be accountable for changing some patterns or habits in our lives, it is best that we join a support group with other people we care about or with those who are facing similar situations.

The Action Here are some basic rules that will help you as you enter any kind of support group situation.

- **Rule 1:** Be yourself! A support group is not a place where you go to make a good impression. You are going there to be cared for, nurtured, and supported.
- **Rule 2:** Attend the same meeting three or four times before making a decision whether it is the right group for you. Try to be an observer the first couple of visits. Save your questions and concerns for someone you trust that might make you feel more comfortable.
- **Rule 3:** Be open to learn from others. It is likely that the people leading a group focusing on losing weight will be recovering from overeating themselves. They can speak from actual

experiences and teach you new tools for coping with your struggles. They can be a great source of encouragement to you.

- **Rule 4:** When attending a group, you are encouraged to talk about yourself and your own experiences. When others share you should listen to what they have to give from their heart. Be careful not to counsel them or give them advice on what they should do.

- **Rule 5:** When using a workbook or other tools in a support group, be sure to stay on schedule with your assignments. Do your best to write your honest feelings in the journal portion of your materials. Use each step to plan for some future choices you want to be held accountable for in the near future.

- **Rule 6:** If codependency is one of the issues you face in your life, be sure that you don't become so focused on the problems of others that you lose sight of your own issues. Try to maintain a balance between caring for others and caring for yourself.

- **Rule 7:** When meeting with a group of people you should maintain confidentiality with regard to what is said. It would be extremely damaging for you to hear one of your personal stories from someone outside the group. And it would be equally damaging for someone else if you shared their story.

- **Rule 8:** Call your sponsor when you are in need of help. If you feel the urge to binge or act in some other destructive way, call for moral support and encouragement. Your sponsor is there for companionship in times of need.

- **Rule 9:** Select your new friends wisely. Some who are not yet healthy may further encourage your addiction to food or may lead you to other addictions. For each friend you establish as part of a group, set up boundaries you are committed to follow when eating together. It's too easy to say things like, "Well, I suppose if we both cheat we'll feel better about it."

- **Rule 10:** Remember daily that you are **not** alone. With the help of God and others you **can** lose weight and recover.

10 SO-SO SODIUM

High sodium diets have been directly linked to high blood pressure, stomach cancer, and strokes.

The Principle Our bodies require that we have a small amount of sodium in our diet every day just as we need a certain amount of protein or other elements. Even some fat is required. However, many people in America are overweight because they take in far too much sodium, protein, and fat in their daily diets. Food by-products are good for us if taken in the right quantities. Taken to extremes, however, certain nutritional items can be dangerous to your health. According to the Pritikin plan we only need 250 to 500 milligrams of sodium per day. This translates into one-fifth of a teaspoon per day.

The Action We recommend that you remove the salt from your table and replace it with a no-salt substitute. Chapter 13 provides some alternative spices for your cooking needs. You will probably find that without salt, the natural flavor of some foods will be enhanced.

Do not assume that any product you buy is low in sodium simply because it is low-calorie. You may be amazed at the quantity of sodium contained in the foods you eat. Try to become more aware of the sodium content of the frozen, canned and other foods you buy at the supermarket. Read the labels very carefully on the products you buy.

Here is a list of some foods that are typically high in sodium content:

packaged frozen and convenience dinners
baked beans
soy sauce
salted nuts
pretzels
frozen waffles
potato chips
bouillon
cooking wine
barbecue and meat sauces
pickles and relishes
salted popcorn
certain canned vegetable juices

chipped beef
hot dogs
processed cheese spreads
olives
canned soups
instant cocoa mixes
catsup
Italian dressing
celery salt
garlic salt
onion salt
smoked fish
bologna
corned beef
sardines
bacon flavored bits
pizza

11 DAILY PERSONAL INVENTORY

Why is it that for many of us the solution to avoiding or dealing with tough emotional days is a pralines and cream double-decker ice cream cone?

The Principle As you continue to read this book you will see that we have purposely intermingled healthy diet ideas with tools for you to get in touch with your emotions. Weight loss is *not* merely a change in diet. In almost every case weight loss involves a change in attitude and outlook.

The Action Do the following exercise to chart how you handle your character weaknesses and how you use your character strengths. Grade yourself in each characteristic using the following scale.

Give yourself a *0* if you are poor at controlling this character weakness or if you do not appropriately display this character strength. Give yourself a *1* if you are fair, a *2* if you are average, a *3* if you think you are good, a *4* if you are great, and a *5* if you are excellent at controlling your behavior in this area.

Common Character Weaknesses

Characteristic	Mon	Tue	Wed	Thu	Fri	Sat	Sun
Anger/ Resentment	___	___	___	___	___	___	___
Approval Seeking	___	___	___	___	___	___	___
Control	___	___	___	___	___	___	___
Denial	___	___	___	___	___	___	___
Depression/ Self-Pity	___	___	___	___	___	___	___
Dishonesty	___	___	___	___	___	___	___
Frozen Feelings	___	___	___	___	___	___	___
Isolation	___	___	___	___	___	___	___
Jealousy	___	___	___	___	___	___	___
Perfectionism	___	___	___	___	___	___	___
Procrastination	___	___	___	___	___	___	___
Worry	___	___	___	___	___	___	___

Common Character Strengths

Characteristic	Mon	Tue	Wed	Thu	Fri	Sat	Sun
Forgiveness	___	___	___	___	___	___	___
Generosity	___	___	___	___	___	___	___
Honesty	___	___	___	___	___	___	___
Humility	___	___	___	___	___	___	___
Patience	___	___	___	___	___	___	___
Risk Taking	___	___	___	___	___	___	___
Self-Control	___	___	___	___	___	___	___
Self-Nurturing	___	___	___	___	___	___	___
Tolerance	___	___	___	___	___	___	___
Trust	___	___	___	___	___	___	___

Areas that are consistently low point to behaviors that you should work on. By focusing on the behaviors, you may be able to avoid the *consequences* of the behaviors—overeating.

12 VACATION SPA

A family each day on their cruise
Were gluttons and then took a snooze
Now they cavort
At a nearby resort
And instead of gaining, they lose

The Principle If vacations are that one time each year when you say, "I'm on vacation. I think I'll eat whatever I want," do you find yourself regretting the way you look and feel when you get home? Plan your vacations carefully, and when you eat, select the foods that will be best for you.

The Action We recommend that you consider vacationing this year at a fitness and nutrition spa or resort. These places are set up to pamper you, help you plan a delicious yet healthy diet, and work with you to set up ways to get in shape.

Most health and fitness resorts are located in beautiful settings throughout the United States. Carefully select a spot that you can afford and that is located in an area where you'd like to travel. Depending on the resort, you can find aerobics, weight training, fitness machines, swimming, tennis, golf, and other athletic activities. In addition, they may offer nutritional lectures and sports evaluations.

- Which sports are you most suited for?
- What muscles in your body are in need of exercise?
- How much body fat do you have?

The instructors can prepare an exercise plan for you to follow the rest of your life. And after exercising, you may want to get a full body massage. What a treat! Many resorts provide full medical examinations to determine the specific diet and vitamins your body most needs.

All meals at health spas are prepared with nutrition in mind. The food is low in calories, fat, and sodium. If you require special meals because of high cholesterol or hypoglycemia, the spa can help you with those needs also.

If you can't afford to go to a spa, plan a vacation where you will focus on good food, exercise, and relaxing fun.

13 ADD A LITTLE SPICE TO YOUR LIFE

Herb and Spice may sound like the names of your neighbors down the street, but they are in essence a couple of kitchen friends that can take the boredom out of dieting.

The Principle As you begin to use ideas from this book and ideas of your own with regard to weight loss, you will want to learn as much as you can about herbs and spices. Dieting is boring to some only because they have not taken the time or energy required to be a little creative with meal preparation.

Generally speaking, spices are hot and herbs are not. Most spices, like sage, ginger, cloves, and mustard, for example, are strongly aromatic, which helps them give food a real bite. Herbs like tarragon, chives, and dill, on the other hand, usually produce a more subtle flavor. Neither spices nor herbs should be used to overpower your meals but rather to enhance them.

The Action One of the first things you may want to do is to buy a book that explains and describes the various herbs and spices used in cooking. Another idea is to enroll in a cooking class targeted at preparing healthy and low-calorie meals. When you are in the supermarket, look at the packaging to learn what spices the big food manufacturers use in their low-calorie meals. As you begin to experiment with herbs and spices, it will be better to use too little rather than using too much.

Be sure to store your herbs and spices in air-tight jars and place them in a cool, dark place. Avoid heat, moisture, and direct sunlight. If you have some old spices around that are more than six months old, you may want to replenish your supply with fresh ingredients.

Here are some hints of various herbs and spices you may want to use on certain foods.

Seasoning Table

Vegetables	*Seasonings*
Broccoli	Dill, mustard seed, tarragon
Carrots	Nutmeg, thyme, ginger, mint, dill, allspice
Peas	Oregano, sage, poppy seed, dill
Potatoes	Celery seed, oregano, thyme, bay leaves
Salads	Basil, dill, tarragon, chives

High Protein Foods

Poultry	Parsley, thyme, sage, marjoram, savory, rosemary

| Meat | Fennel, bay leaves, sage, savory, tarragon, thyme |
| Fish | Bay leaves, dill, fennel, marjoram, rosemary, thyme |

Ethnic Foods

Chinese	Ginger, hot mustard, garlic, curry, cayenne
Indian	Garlic, saffron, turmeric, cumin, cinnamon
Mexican	Chile powder, oregano, cumin, chile pepper flakes
Italian	Garlic, sweet basil, fennel, rosemary, marjoram, oregano

14 A MIGHTY METABOLISM

Perhaps you have been eating more healthy and lower calorie meals without seeing great amounts of weight loss. While losing weight requires less of ingredients such as fatty foods it may require more of one ingredient— aerobic exercise.

The Principle Some people find it harder than others to lose weight despite the fact that they may have greatly improved their diet. When you eat less, your body automatically adjusts its metabolism to a lower level. This can often leave you feeling tired, grumpy, and hungry. Perhaps you need to find ways to raise your metabolism.

The Action The best way to raise your metabolism while you diet is through regular aerobic exercise—walking, running, biking, rowing, and dancing or exercise classes.

As you exercise, your body replaces fat tissue with muscle tissue, which further increases your body's caloric consumption and helps with weight loss. Fat is reduced and your metabolism works more efficiently to keep you in shape.

Here are some things to consider when you are making your plan for aerobic exercise.

- *Make exercise an absolute way of life.* Consider your daily exercise to be as routine as brushing your teeth, eating, setting your alarm or showering. You may have to force yourself to exercise regularly at first, but after a while, it will become routine.
- *Schedule your exercise time appropriately.* If you already find it difficult to get out of bed each morning, it doesn't make much sense to set your exercise time for five o'clock in the morning. Instead, find a way to exercise during your lunch hour or after you get home at the end of the day.
- *Find other benefits to your exercise.* Perhaps you love the outdoors. Consider your daily exercise another opportunity to go outside and run, walk, and bike along your favorite beach or park.
- *Don't overdue it at first.* If you have selected running as your aerobic exercise and you have not run in ten years, begin by running only a few blocks during the first week. In week two, run twice that distance. Set a schedule for gradual increases as time goes on.
- *Seek guidance in your exercise.* Consider joining a health club near your home or work. In most cases the club will design a program that will be tailored to your needs. You might even want to join the club with a family member or friend to encourage each other in attendance and regular workouts.
- *Enjoy your exercise through music.* If you find

exercise tough, consider getting headphones and tape player so that you can listen to your favorite music as you jog, bike, or work out.

- *Buy some workout clothes.* Consider enrolling in some aerobic classes near your home. But before you go, shop for some workout clothes that make you look good. If you look good to yourself as you exercise, you will probably be encouraged.
- *Make your first plan.* In the spaces below, briefly outline your first steps in creating an aerobic exercise plan.

Aerobic Exercise Plan

Possible friends/companions I can exercise with

_____

_____

WEEK 1

Starting date _____

Type of exercise _____

Length of time I will exercise each
   day _____

Time of day I will begin
   exercising _____

WEEK 2

Starting date _____
Type of exercise _____
Length of time I will exercise each
   day _____
Time of day I will begin
   exercising _____

WEEK 3

Starting date _____
Type of exercise _____
Length of time I will exercise each
   day _____
Time of day I will begin
   exercising _____

15 SAY NO TO SODAS

Have you ever heard anyone say, "Ever since I've been drinking diet cola I've lost thirty pounds"? Probably not.

The Principle Over 200 million soft drinks are consumed every year in this country. Aside from the ingredients that can add unwanted weight, which we will discuss further, soft drinks can be harmful to your body in other ways. Dr. Clive McCay of Cornell University showed that soft drinks can completely erode tooth enamel and make teeth soft in a very short time.

The malic acids and citric acids found in fruits and vegetables turn alkaline in the body's system. Though soft drinks contain malic acids, they also contain carbonic acid, phosphoric acid, erythorbic acid, and other acids that do *not* turn alkaline. The pH balance in your system is thrown off course with the first sip of these acids.

The Action Instead of drinking various sodas, begin drinking sparkling water, herbal tea, or some other healthy substitute. The typical soft drink has refined white sugar—about five teaspoons per eight-ounce serving.

If you think that drinking diet sodas will be a major factor in dropping those unwanted pounds, you may be misleading yourself. As awful as this may sound, diet soft drinks taken with food cause your food to ferment or rot in your stomach instead of digesting. The diet soda prevents the food from being broken down in an efficient manner, thereby requiring more energy from your body to digest a normal low-calorie meal.

Diet sodas also contain high amounts of sodium, which leads to water retention. Many also contain caffeine, which is an addictive substance. Our society somehow has equated diet drinks with healthy drinks. This is not necessarily the case.

16 DAY BY DAY

It's when you look behind at the failures of the past or ahead at the worries of the future that life becomes tough. Real peace comes through celebrating the precious blessing of each present moment God gives to us.

The Principle One of the secrets to life is learning to make decisions on a day-to-day basis rather than tackling a year-long or life-long project. Recovery from any behavior or pattern requires that choices be made one day at a time. As we go through life we make millions of choices—some good for us, some bad for us. If you can start today with some good choices and continue that each new day, over time you will find that many old bad habits have been changed into new good ones.

The Action Here are some one-day-at-a-time choices you can make that will change your life.

- *On this day* . . . I will try to be happy. My happiness is a direct result of my being at peace with myself; what others do or think will not determine my happiness.
- *On this day* . . . I will accept myself and live to the best of my ability.
- *On this day* . . . I will make time to pray and meditate on the Scriptures, seeking God and developing my relationship with Him.

- *On this day* . . . I say what I mean and mean what I say.
- *On this day* . . . I will make healthy choices to eat food that will help me nutritionally and that will help me reach my goals.
- *On this day* . . . I will not tackle all my problems at once but live moment to moment at my very best.
- *On this day* . . . I will live my life being assertive, not aggressive; being humble, not proud; being confident to be exactly who I am.
- *On this day* . . . I will take care of my physical health. I will exercise my mind, my body, and my spirit.
- *On this day* . . . I will be kind to those around me. I will be agreeable, finding no fault with others. Nor will I try to improve or regulate others.
- *On this day* . . . I will remind myself that God has a special place in His heart for me and a special purpose for me to fill in this world.

17 ON A PRAYER

I can do all things through Christ who strengthens me.—Philippians 4:13

The Principle When we are too weak emotionally or spiritually to face a major challenge, the God who created us tells us that we can do all things through Him. Spiritual growth with our Lord is not something that comes overnight. Rather, as we put our trust in Him day after day, month after month, year after year, we grow to love Him and know that He really does encourage us when we are down. Regular prayer focusing on our weaknesses and encouraging scriptures like the one above give us the power to do all things through Him.

The Action Through prayer and meditation, improve your conscious contact with God. Ask for His will for your life and for the power to make the dramatic changes. Putting it simply, Colossians 3:16 says, "Let the word of Christ dwell in you richly."

By spending time with God you can learn that you are His treasured gift. Once you realize how valuable you are, your self-esteem will grow. You will find yourself with a new power to overcome obstacles to your weight loss—whether they be bad eating habits or painful emotions.

Your self-esteem will grow as you make God your trusted friend, and prayer is the best way to build that relationship.

- Ask to be kept free from self-pity, dishonesty, and selfishness.
- Ask to be guided as you face the problems in your life.
- Ask that His will be done each day.
- Pray to be forgiven when you have hurt others or yourself.
- Thank Him for the love He has shown you.
- Ask that He reveal Himself to you each day.
- Turn to Him instead of turning to food for comfort.
- Ask that He satisfy your desires with good things.
- Ask that He allow you to be a vessel of His love for others.
- Ask to have peace within your heart.
- Ask to be more like Him each day.
- Ask that your faith in Him grow and that your relationship will nourish a growing self-esteem.

18 AEROBIC DANCING

And one and two and three and four!

The Principle For those who find regular jogging boring or who do not have access to a swimming pool, aerobic dancing can have a twofold benefit: it is a great way to get into shape, tone your body, and lose weight; and it is fun. Aerobic dancing is a combination of rhythmic movements and simple steps set to music that can improve and maintain cardiovascular and physical fitness. The American Heart Association supports aerobic dancing.

The Action As with other types of exercise, be careful to start off slowly. Don't overdo it at first, and always stretch your muscles before and after exercising. Begin with a low-impact program—especially if you have knee or back problems. If you feel out of breath, take it easy for a while, jog slowly in place or maintain regular steady movements.

- Ideally, an aerobic dance program begins with a warm-up period to increase respiration, circulation, and body temperature.

- The actual aerobic dancing that follows should last for twenty to thirty minutes.
- The program should then end with a cool-down period. After a few months, you will find yourself out of breath less often and your endurance will be increased.

Most health clubs around the country offer regular classes for people at all levels. Or you can purchase one of the work-out videotapes on the market.

Aerobic dancing is a great activity to do with a friend so that you encourage each other to work out regularly. Be careful not to become competitive, however. Everyone is different and handles various types of exercise in a unique way to others. If your friend can do all 300 sit-ups and you can't, it's okay. Perhaps he or she is in better shape than you. The goal is for *you* to lose weight and tone your body, not for you to out-jump your friend.

If you find yourself losing weight after attending classes and eating better for a certain length of time, *don't stop!* This is the very time you need to continue your exercise to further tone up your body and keep the weight off. Once someone who exercises regularly stops their activity, the benefits gained from the exercise are lost rapidly.

19 BUDDY, BUDDY

In the Old Testament book of Ecclesiastes, it says that, "Two are better than one, because they have a good reward for their labor. For if they fall, one will lift up his companion. But woe to him who is alone when he falls, for he has no one to help him up." (Ecclesiastes 4:9–10)

The Principle If you have a spouse, roommate, or friend who needs to lose weight too, use the buddy system to encourage each other, provide accountability, and celebrate victories.

The Action Find someone with a similar goal to be your buddy while you lose the weight and for the months afterward when you commit to keeping it off.

The Planning Meeting

Start with a planning meeting to discuss what your goals will be and how you plan on working together to achieve your goals. It is good to talk about how difficult it is to be overweight and how it is affecting your life. Prior to getting together you may want to each fill out the following information and then share it with one another during your planning meeting.

1. My weight problem affects my life in the following ways:

2. I find myself eating other than at mealtime for the following reasons:

3. I would like to lose _____ pounds in _____ months.
4. I am committing myself to reach this goal by _____ [date].
5. I further commit to helping _____ _____ achieve his/her goal by providing encouragement and support.

_____   _____
Signature   Date

Restock the Kitchen

Together go through all of the cupboards and the refrigerators in your house(s) and give or throw away all food that is fattening or causes you to overeat. Sit down together to plan your shopping list of healthy foods, and then go to the store together and buy only those items on your list. Set up times for the two of you to meet regularly and track your plans.

Set up an Exercise Plan

In addition to planning your food intake, plan regular times to exercise together. Not only will you be furthering your efforts to lose weight, you will probably have fun exercising with your mate or buddy. Perhaps you will even strengthen your relationship or friendship.

Start to get in good shape by walking early in the morning for about fifteen minutes. After a week, increase your walk to thirty minutes and after another week to forty-five minutes. As you increase your time, also increase your pace. Walking is an aerobic exercise that can shed inches off of your body, strengthen your heart, and suppress your appetite. Your metabolism and energy should increase.

Stay in Touch Daily

Develop, as part of your plan, a way to call one another throughout the day for encouragement and support. Once you've met your goals, plan a maintenance program to help keep the weight off.

20 THE FATS OF THE MATTER

They don't call them fats for nothing!

The Principle Much of the food we eat is filled with fats, which, when consumed contribute to the percentage of fat make-up of our body chemistry. Each time you eat, if you are able to greatly reduce the fat content of your meals, you will greatly reduce the amount of fats flowing through your system. For example, let's look at the fat content of a typical meal.

Beef Stroganoff

Ingredients	Calories
Two tablespoons of margarine	200
One pound of sirloin steak	951
One clove of garlic	4
One and a half cups of chopped mushrooms	27
One half cup of chopped onion	27
One tablespoon of flour	25
Eight ounces of sour cream	416
One ten-and-a-half ounce can of mushroom soup	313
Two cups of hot cooked noodles	400
Total calories	2,363

Calories per serving	591
Grams of fat per serving	29

The Action   Instead of preparing foods that are higher in both calories and fat, consider replacing meals like the one above with entrees that are healthier. Your Beef Stroganoff could be replaced with the following entree. Compare the two entrees. Not only does the substitute dish contain fewer than half the calories, the fat-gram content drops a great deal from twenty-nine to four. Imagine what would happen if you did this at every meal!

Vegetable/Pasta Stroganoff

Ingredients	*Calories*
Four cups of vegetables	300
One clove of garlic	4
One and one half cups of chopped mushrooms	27
Two tablespoons of flour	50
One cup of evaporated milk	200
One package of instant onion soup mix	35
Eight ounces of plain, nonfat yogurt	100
Two cups of pasta (cooked)	400
Total calories	1,116
Calories per serving	279
Grams of fat per serving	4

Cooking instructions: In a saucepan sprayed with a low-calorie, nonstick oil, stir-fry all the bite-sized vegetables and garlic. Add the mushrooms just before the other vegetables are fully cooked.

In another pan, prepare the sauce. Add the flour to the evaporated milk and stir until the flour dissolves. Mix these ingredients with the instant mushroom soup in a medium saucepan over medium heat, stirring constantly until boiling. Add the yogurt and stir to a simmer. Combine the sauce with the vegetables and pasta.

21 AM I REALLY HUNGRY?

Sometimes we eat to satisfy a hunger that may be for something other than food!

The Principle The course of action we take when the urge to eat overwhelms us can serve as a sort of barometer to measure our general state of health and well-being. If we eat because of the right reasons, the "well-being barometer" tells us it's okay. If we eat when we don't really need to, the barometer can be telling us something is wrong.

The Action Before you eat, ask yourself if you are really hungry or are you heading toward the refrigerator for some other reason? Consider the following as answers you might have to this question.

- *I'm really hungry!* Let's get the obvious one out of the way first. You may have a genuine, legitimate need for food. After all, it is a natural human function to require nourishment. You had no choice in that decision. The amounts and kinds of foods you eat to satisfy that requirement are choices you make for yourself.

  You can take responsibility for changing your patterns. That's what the ideas in this book are all about. If you don't know what your body needs to remain healthy, consult a physician or nutritionist for proper guidelines.

Even if you don't overeat, consuming the wrong foods moderately can cause weight gain and can adversely affect your health. Education about the right foods, nutritional counseling, and your ability to stick to a plan can be the keys to healthy eating when hunger strikes.

- *I'm not really hungry. Perhaps my body could use some exercise or rest.* Consider the option of exercise. If you can't find the time to exercise, try changing your schedule so that you go to bed an hour earlier so you get up in time to do a light workout. The time to exercise will always exist if you move it from the bottom of your priorities to a place near the top!

  You don't have to join the local health club to exercise. Consider running in place. Take a vigorous walk. Work out with an aerobics video on the VCR! Just think what would happen if once a day you exercised, if only for a short while, instead of taking one of your trips to the kitchen.

- *I'm not really hungry. I'm eating because I'm feeling lonely.* Perhaps you are using food to fill an emotional need. But using food to replace some emotional void can lead to disaster. If you are eating because you are lonely, find some other way to deal with the hurt. Consider getting professional help if the problem continues. Food will never meet your emotional needs, but it *can* bring you down to a state of guilt and remorse.

- *I'm not really hungry. I'm eating because I'm angry and afraid.* Like loneliness, feelings such as anger over past experiences or fear of future uncertainties can draw you to food. You actually may be medicating your problem with food rather than attempting to heal the pain.

Consider finding a therapist to help you answer the question of why you escape the pain by turning to food. You may be able to free yourself of some past hurts and find out who you *really* are. Perhaps you can join a support group in your area where you can feel safe in sharing your feelings with others in similar situations.

22 HOLIDAY LIGHTS

The night before Christmas was still,
with no sounds
But we ate all the goodies and gained
a few pounds

The Principle Holidays are notorious for eating, more eating, and still more eating. Often the good cheer is replaced with heartburn, that bloated feeling and ten pounds of excess baggage. The constant presence of fudge, holiday cookies, candy eggs, and office parties present us with more temptation to overeat unhealthy foods than at other times throughout the year.

The Action Give yourself and your family a special gift of nutrition this year by implementing some of the following tips to keep from turning a season of joy to a season of blues. Often, the holidays are the toughest times of the year for the overeater because the focus is turned from the reason for the season to the pain of the gain.

Here are a few tips that might help you during holidays such as Easter, Thanksgiving, and Christmas where high-calorie foods are much more plentiful.

- Leave the gravy off your turkey and other foods of your holiday meals.

- Replace the potatoes and the stuffing with creative, vegetable side dishes.
- Implement some of the lower-calorie dessert items mentioned in this book (low-calorie cheesecake, cinnamon rolls, and hot apple crunch) rather than the traditional pies and tarts eaten during holiday periods.
- Pass on the chocolates you receive as gifts to a family in need or business associates—but give them to people who don't struggle with overeating or weight problems.
- Replace the typical Easter basket filled of high-calorie goodies with a traditional, health-food basket. Include items such as granola bars, unsalted almonds, dried fancy fruits, and sugar-free candies.
- For the kids' Easter egg hunt, use plastic eggs in which you can place prizes, small toys, or money.
- For hors d'oeuvres, make fruit salads and vegetable platters.
- Consider giving up alcohol and replacing it with hot apple cider. For a special treat add cinnamon and nutmeg. Replace other high-calorie beverages such as eggnog with flavored nonfat yogurt shakes.
- Since ham is very high in both fat and sodium, replace it with roast chicken.
- Instead of stuffing the stockings with lots of candies and goodies, use small gifts such as matchbox cars, barrettes, and certificates for nights at the movies.

23 I SAID RELAX, NOT RELAPSE

If you have built castles in the air, your work need not be lost; that is where they should be. Now put the foundations under them.

—Thoreau

The Principle Setting up principles to avoid relapse from the early stages can help you prevent future relapses. What does the term *relapse* mean when it comes to food? Relapse occurs for over-eaters whenever we slip off the path and eat food that is not on our plan or when we stop exercising according to the plan we've established.

Normally when we relapse, there were things that happened prior to the slip that caused us to make bad decisions. If we become aware of these events we can avoid a relapse the next time by refusing to eat the wrong foods or to let go of our exercise.

The Action Here are some questions you should ask yourself if you feel you are about to slip or relapse:

- Do you find yourself being obsessed with food, cookbooks, and recipes or being overly preoccupied with food in general?
- Are you isolating more—pulling back from your support group, buddy, or healthy relationship?
- Are you gaining weight and unaware of how this is happening?
- Are you rationalizing all the reasons to go off your diet and telling yourself you don't need to eat the right foods? Are you saying things like, "I'm weak because I haven't eaten enough food" or "I can do this thing my own way?"
- Are you finding new ways to keep so busy that you're not exercising?
- Are you aware of resentment or anger building that you are not working through or resolving?

If you find that you answered yes to one or more of the above questions, if you have just relapsed, or if you feel a relapse coming, here are some suggestions to get back on track.

- *Forgive yourself.* Be kind and compassionate with yourself. You are human and therefore not perfect. Review with yourself the valuable lessons that you learned from this experience and how you can make positive changes from it that will affect the rest of your life.
- *Share your problem with a friend.* Confession is a powerful healer. If you don't ask a friend to

help you, you'll probably keep emotionally beating yourself up.

- *Inventory the steps that led to your relapse.* This will be of great value for you in the future. Create a list of warning signs that you can watch for in the future to catch relapses in their early stages.
- *Write out a script.* Plan how you would react if the same situation arose again. Use this script to develop a new strategy.
- *Get back on your path.* Exercise even when you don't feel like it. Begin again to eat healthy foods.

24 BUT I'M IN A HURRY

If you always eat on the run
A greasy hamburger and bun
Eat other foods
Or else your bad moods
Will worsen as you reach a ton

The Principle Fast-food restaurants can be habit forming. And many of the people who eat there claim that, "It's the only place I could get a quick meal." But believe us, you can break your fast-food habit, eat alternative foods, or find a fast-food restaurant that offers healthy choices as part of their menu.

The Action Here are some suggestions for alternative food to eat when you are on the run.

- Instead of running into the donut shop, stop at the grocery store and pick up some low-fat yogurt and a piece of fruit.
- When you must go to a fast-food restaurant, select one that offers a salad bar or grilled chicken sandwiches.
- Pack a small cooler in your trunk, especially if you're going on the road. Fill the cooler with

carrot sticks, celery sticks, nonfat yogurt, fruit, and a salad for lunch.

- On your day off prepare meals for the week. Some ideas include roasted chicken breasts and stir-fried vegetables. Put the items that are able to be frozen into freezer bags in one-meal portions and freeze them. Each day, pull out a well-prepared meal for yourself and heat it in the oven or microwave. Or, if you are on the road, pull out a meal that will taste good even if it is just thawed rather than cooked.
- Buy a small refrigerator for your office. When you have evening meetings on your way home from work and only a small amount of time to eat, avoid the temptation of stopping for an unhealthy meal by storing your dinner in this refrigerator. Eat your dinner before you leave for your meeting.
- When you stop by a convenience store, purchase things like unsalted almonds and unsweetened fruit juice rather than cupcakes and soft drinks.
- Pack a supply of protein powder in your office and trunk along with plenty of water in your cooler.
- Keep a supply of no-salt or low-salt broth mixes near you for a quick and filling snack.
- Have a supply of cans containing low-fat, low-salt tuna fish and chicken breast stored in your office and trunk. Also, keep a can opener, pa-

per plates, napkins, and utensils handy for such quick meals.
- Find other ideas in this book that talk about low-calorie recipes that you can store for quick meals.

25 HALF EMPTY OR HALF FULL?

Perhaps it dates back to the days when parents said, "You cannot leave the table until your plate is empty." So today we eat everything on our plate after we've already gone back for seconds! The only thing stuffed at a meal should be a cabbage or tomato—not you!

The Principle Perhaps you have tried to lose weight by missing meals altogether. One of the problems with this is that when we deprive ourselves of food during one mealtime, we often overdo our eating during the next mealtime. When you break from a regular eating routine, you may find yourself unable to determine when you are full.

The Action Make sure you are *physically* hungry before you eat. If you are starving for affection, affirmation, attention, or love, and turn to food, you will never feel full because food cannot satisfy those feelings of emptiness. And you'll just keep eating because food only satisfies physical hunger, not emotional hunger.

When it is time to eat a meal, think about what you are going to eat before you actually sit down or begin to prepare it. If you leave your choices to impulse and don't make a specific decision, chances are you will eat things that are not good for you. When making your plan, think of healthy foods that you enjoy. If you select something that is boring, you may find yourself eating something else after you've completed your healthy meal. Obviously, this is to be avoided. Allow yourself to enjoy the food's texture, temperature, and ingredients.

Begin today to pay close attention to how *much* you eat. Teach yourself when to know that enough is enough. Start by asking yourself after every meal, "Do I feel comfortably satisfied or uncomfortably full?" Perhaps you could rank how you feel on a scale from one to ten, five being the ideal level of comfort and ten being so full you can hardly move from the table. (We've all been there.)

Think in your recent past of some meals you've had where you felt comfortable but not completely full. Visualize how large the portion of food was. Describe that meal and the portion size below.

Recent meal where I felt comfortable, not full

_____

_____

As you look toward the future, start documenting each meal with the one-to-ten ranking system. This will help you decide how large the portions of food you should target for future meals. Here is a chart to plot your next several meals.

Meal Portions and Comfort Ranking

Meal and Date	Food Eaten	Portion Size	1 to 10 Com- fort Ranking
_____	_____	_____	_____
_____	_____	_____	_____
_____	_____	_____	_____
_____	_____	_____	_____
_____	_____	_____	_____
_____	_____	_____	_____
_____	_____	_____	_____
_____	_____	_____	_____

If you are finding that you feel uncomfortably full (a ranking of eight or more) after many of your meals, set a goal for your next meal to finish with a ranking of four or five. This is just one more step that will help you take control and remain in control of the quantity of food you eat.

26 DESERT DESSERT

There once was a man named Lloyd
Whose chocolate he could not avoid
But now he abstains
And so he remains
Much thinner and lots less annoyed

The Principle If you are fifteen to twenty pounds overweight and do not overeat, perhaps you should analyze what makes up your diet. Do you eat dessert after many or most evening meals? Is it difficult for you to refrain from eating chocolate when you're near it? If you answer yes to these types of questions, it should be quite obvious that your extra weight is not caused by how much you eat—but by *what* you are eating. Desserts and other sweets cause thousands and thousands of extra calories and excess fat to your diet over several months' time.

The Action There are lots of ways you can cut down on the desserts and other sweets you eat. You may choose to give up chocolate if you eat it quite a bit. That will still allow you to eat other desserts occasionally. Or perhaps you eat far too much ice cream now and want to make a commitment to eat it only on very special occasions.

Try sharing your dessert with a spouse or friend. Or try eating dessert just one night a week. You also could switch to desserts that are lower in calories. When invited to a dinner party, offer to bring your own low-calorie dessert for everyone to share.

Here are a few suggestions for desserts that you may want to eat in moderation as long as you continue to exercise and follow the rest of the plan you have made.

apple pie, sugarless
cappuccino
fruit salad, unsweetened
gelatin, sugarless
ice milk
peaches and nonfat milk
popcorn, unsalted and unbuttered
raisins and granola
sherbet
strawberries, fresh
vanilla wafers
yogurt, nonfat and sugarless

If sugar affects your system a great deal, it will be important to check first with a doctor and then wean yourself from the large quantity of sugar you eat. Immediate sugar voids for some people can cause withdrawal symptoms such as headaches, dizziness, and a loss of energy. But as your system adjusts as you begin to eat more healthy foods, you will probably find you have more energy than ever before.

After a time of weaning yourself away from desserts with the most fats, you may be able to say good-bye to all desserts. Chances are you will notice a great deal of weight loss if you previously were used to eating a lot of sugar and fat-filled treats.

27 A TRIP TO THE SALAD BAR

Many well-intentioned people who really want to lose weight opt for the salad bar only to pile more calories on top of their lettuce than are found in a hot fudge sundae!

The Principle   Much of the population has the false belief that "if it is part of the salad bar setup, it must be a low-calorie food." This is not necessarily the case in many salad bars today—even in the finest restaurants. Some people even feel that since it's only salad they can go back for as many trips as possible and still stay remarkably thin.

The Action   If you are unable to eat foods in moderate portions, buffet-style and all-you-can-eat salad bar restaurants are not safe places for you to dine. Set your food limit with regard to quantity and then stick to it. If certain kinds of restaurants tempt you to eat too much food or the wrong food, stay away from them.

Many soup and salad restaurants serve delicious foods. But some of the items served include such moderate to high-calorie foods as creamed soups, pasta salads, and freshly-baked muffins topped with three different types of butter. Creamed soups are loaded with calories, carbohydrates, sodium, and fats. Pasta salads contain massive amounts of mayonnaise at 100 high-fat calories per tablespoon. The muffins contain a great deal of sugar, and the butter will add another 100 high-fat calories per level tablespoon.

Fortunately, these restaurants also have all the foods our bodies need to stay on a well-planned food program. We only need to use care when making our selections.

- Build your salad with lettuce, beets, tomatoes, cucumbers, beans, sprouts, onions, peas, and any other fresh vegetables.
- When you get to the salad dressing, go easy. Remember that mayonnaise is extremely high in fat and calories. Vinegar and oil dressing is good in moderation. But lemon slices squeezed over the salad is even better. A compromise would be to combine a small quantity of a low-calorie dressing with a few lemon slices.
- Avoid the soup entirely. Because of the high salt content, it's just not worth the joy of consumption.
- If the bread department has freshly baked squaw bread, have one piece, but do not add butter.
- For your beverage have some iced or hot herbal tea or mineral water.

Skip the dessert bar altogether. Chances are, if you made your salad from the proper foods and ate your piece of bread, you will be sufficiently full. Practice making healthy salads to show yourself that **you** can control the food rather than having the **food** control you!

28 A LITTLE EXERCISE NEVER HURT

In addition to a regular exercise routine, you can do little things each day to burn off a few extra calories.

The Principle Losing weight can be accomplished best through a combination of different actions that include making changes to your eating patterns, revising the way you face your emotions, and starting a routine of regular exercise. But you can do little things each and every day to help get and keep yourself fit.

The Action Here are some practical things you can do every day to burn off those few extra calories. Many modern conveniences have made it easy for us to take short cuts, and the more short cuts we take the easier it is to gain a pound or two. As a general rule, when you go from one place to another, figure out a way that you can arrive at your destination using more aerobics and less automation.

- Use the stairs instead of the elevator. Set a rule for yourself that any time you are going up or down fewer than five floors, you take the stairs,

- If you take the bus, train, or subway to work or school, don't board it at the closest stop to your home. Instead, make it a habit to walk to a stop twenty to thirty minutes away.
- If it is practical, ride your bike to work instead of taking a car or other transportation. If this is not practical, ride your bike or walk on errands or when going to the market.
- Take an exercise break instead of a coffee break. Keep a pair of tennis shoes at your office and walk around the block a couple of times.
- Leave your car parked at the furthest end of a parking lot and walk vigorously to your destination. Walk completely around a mall before you start shopping.
- While at home watching television, ride an exercise bike or rowing machine. If you don't have one, do 10 sit-ups during every commercial break of some one-hour program you watch. Build up to 20 sit-ups, then 30, and finally 50.
- While doing simple chores around your home, wear ankle and wrist weights.
- Next time you have to drive the kids to work, band practice, or Little League, walk them there instead.
- Perhaps there is no way you can find fifty minutes a day for regular exercise, so do the next best thing. Find five ten-minute intervals

throughout the day to get your exercising done.

- Set your alarm fifteen minutes early each day and take a short walk to a special place near your home.

29 SAY CHEESE-CAKE

You may choose to stay on a very strict diet, giving up desserts altogether. On the other hand, if you have exercised regularly, eaten the right foods at each meal, and have seen your weight drop, you can still serve desserts as long as you find ways to cut down on the high-fat, high-calorie ingredients.

The Principle By replacing traditional ingredients in a dessert such as cheesecake with items lower in fats and calories, you can make delicious treats to serve at special meals. For example, sour cream can be omitted with no loss of flavor. And whipped egg whites will create a more delicate cheesecake as well as providing one that is more healthy than one using the entire egg. Use light cream cheese, yogurt, and low-fat cottage cheese to replace regular cream cheese. Although your dessert will still contain about 200 calories per slice, the typical cheesecake has almost 600 per serving.

The Action Here is a cheesecake recipe we hope you'll enjoy making and eating. Remember, just because it is lower in calories doesn't mean you can eat this treat as a meal. Serve it to your guests and yourself in small tasty portions.

Strawberry Cheesecake

vegetable cooking spray
1/4 cup vanilla wafer crumbs
  (about 28 small cookies)
1 (24 oz.) carton 1 percent low-
  fat cottage cheese
2 (8 oz.) tubs light process
  cream cheese
1 cup sugar
2 eggs

4 egg whites
1/8 teaspoon cream of tartar
2 3/4 cups halved fresh
  strawberries
strawberry topping (optional—
  purée 2 cups fresh
  strawberries in a blender and
  pour over cheesecake)

Coat the bottom of a 10-inch springform pan with cooking spray; sprinkle with cookie crumbs and set aside.

Blend together the cottage cheese and cream cheese until smooth. Add 3/4 cup sugar, and 2 whole eggs; blend until smooth. Pour into a large bowl and set aside.

Beat 4 egg whites (at room temperature) and cream of tartar at high speed with an electric mixer until foamy. Gradually add the remaining 1/4 cup of sugar, one tablespoon at a time, beating until stiff peaks form.

Gently stir one-fourth of egg white mixture into cream cheese mixture and fold in remaining egg whites.

Pour the mixture into the prepared pan. Bake at 325° for 50 minutes. Remove pan from oven. Cool for 15 minutes. Cover and chill at least eight hours.

Add strawberries to top of the cheesecake. Drizzle with strawberry glaze.

30 FOR GENER- ATIONS TO COME

Much of who we are and what we've become has been shaped by the environment and people who were around us as we were children. And we have the ability to change the next generation.

The Principle We have been influenced to a great extent by the people who raised us and the environment that surrounded us. Some of those influences were wonderful and helped mold us into the good people we are. And some may have been bad influences or habits that caused a lack of proper emotional or physical health within us. We have at least two choices how we can deal with those bad habits and pains. We can either blame those who we think were responsible or we can forgive them and take responsibility for changing the unhealthy or unlikable parts of ourselves.

But beyond that, we can have a great influence over the children currently in our lives so that they can grow up with healthier habits and happier memories. Begin now to teach your kids that proper eating and regular exercise is important to growing into healthy adults.

The Action   If your weight problem is caused by bad eating habits you learned from your parents or from some unresolved emotional pain, don't let history repeat itself. Bring your children up with good eating habits and seek professional help to see how you can avoid passing on family dysfunction to your kids.

Begin your assessment by asking these questions regarding your children.

- Are your children within the average weight range for their heights?
- Do your children engage in some sort of active play such as tag, basketball, bike riding, ballet, or jogging every day for at least an hour?
- Do your children participate in daily gym classes at school?
- Do you participate with your children in physical activities such as walking, swimming, hiking, or cycling?
- Do your children spend less than two hours watching television or reading each day?
- Do you encourage your children to eat fresh fruits, vegetables, whole grain breads, and low-fat dairy products?
- Do you discourage your children from eating hot dogs, hamburgers, french fries, chips, and ice cream on a regular basis?
- Do you know your children's cholesterol levels?
- Do you limit your children's consumption of chocolate, cookies, and other sweets?

- Do you teach your children the importance of balanced meals and regular exercise?

If you answered no to several questions, chances are that your children are not growing up as healthy as they could. Perhaps it is time you help your children begin developing healthy eating habits and teach them to spend less time on the couch.

31 A FAMILY AFFAIR

Work together as a family to help one another become more healthy.

The Principle Involve the entire family in the effort to lose weight, to exercise, and to change some bad habits. Make fitness a family affair.

The Action

Hold a Family Meeting.

Begin your new efforts by holding a family meeting. Discuss why you want to help one another become more healthy. Talk about weight loss, increased energy, and a higher self-esteem. Ask what new activities the family would like to learn together. Encourage one another to eat healthy meals when away from one another at work or school.

Set a Schedule.

Set aside regular times each week to work out together, rescheduling mealtimes or homework if necessary. If the entire family cannot always exercise as a group, each person could pair up with another.

Motivate One Another.

You may even need to help one another with chores around the house so that everyone will have time to be involved. Set goals, chart your progress, and give awards when goals are reached.

Weekend Plans.

Make plans in advance to do special things like bike rides or nature hikes on the weekends. Go on picnics together featuring healthy, low-calorie meals.

Mealtime.

Discuss as a family which foods are good to eat and which are unhealthy or full of fat. If you don't eat many meals together now, do everything you can to arrange more meals together. If you have an especially creative and close family, schedule different family members to cook throughout the week!

Documentation.

Keep a family journal of the goals you set, the activities you do, and the ideas you generate. Take pictures regularly to document your activities and to show the progress you've made.

Ask for Further Help.

Ask that God will give you the strength and will-power to get over the hurdles, change old patterns, and reach new goals.

32 HOSTESS WITH THE LEASTEST

Just because you want to lose weight doesn't mean you have to give up all the social events in your life that center around food. You can help your friends lose weight too!

The Principle The majority of our social time with others is centered around eating. Those times can be equally as fun and relationship-building if we ensure that the foods we eat are healthy and low in calories. In fact, we will probably be around for many more years of socializing if we take more care in eating the right foods.

The Action Host regular low-calorie dinner parties for your family and friends. Your temptation may be to use the everyday dishes just because you are holding back on the calories. Instead, bring out your best china and invite friends over for a meal, whether or not they, too, struggle with weight problems. Here is a sample menu for your dinner of four.

Vegetable salad with your own house dressing
Roast chicken breast
Roasted potatoes and vegetables
Baked apple crunch

Sparkling mineral water with lemon slices
Iced herbal tea

Vegetable Salad

1 1/2 heads of lettuce	1 tomato
1 cucumber peeled and thinly sliced	2 shredded carrots
	Bean sprouts

Serve with your "house" dressing. (Add one part low-fat milk to three parts of your favorite low calorie cream-style dressing—this further reduces the calories per serving.)

Roast Chicken Breasts with Roasted Potatoes and Vegetables

4 large skinned chicken breasts	8 sliced fresh carrots
4 large white rose potatoes	1 8 oz. bottle of reduced calorie Italian dressing
1 head broccoli	1/4 cup diet margarine
1 onion	2 tablespoons no-salt seasoning
1 clove crushed garlic	

In a large roasting pan, put thinly-sliced (1/4 inch) white rose potatoes to form the bottom layer. Next, place equally thin-sliced carrots to form a second layer. Sprinkle garlic and no-salt seasoning and 1/4 bottle of the dressing. Next, lay the four large chicken breasts on the vegetables. Add one sliced onion. Cover with the broccoli in large pieces, stems removed. Pour on the rest of the bottle of salad dressing. Sprinkle evenly the rest of the garlic and more no-salt seasoning along with the margarine. Cover and bake at 350° for one hour.

(Vegetarians can still create a delicious meal by leaving out the chicken.)

Hot Apple Crunch

1 jar (24 oz.) unsweetened
applesauce (contains no
sugar)

1/2 bag of cinnamon special
granola

Bake applesauce at 350° until boiling hot. Spoon into your favorite dessert goblets a layer of applesauce and then a layer of granola. Continue alternating layers until you reach the top of your goblets. Be sure to finish with a layer of granola on top.

33 BALLROOM BOOGIE

Ballroom dancing can elevate your heart rate as much as running or cross-country skiing.

The Principle   Recent surveys have shown ballroom dancing to be one of the best exercises. You can burn up to 400 calories per hour dancing.

The Action   Sign up either on your own or with your mate for a ballroom dancing class. In addition to learning a new social activity, ballroom dancing will help you tone your entire body. As part of the instruction you will learn many different dances and dance steps. Swings and polkas are especially excellent for burning fat and toning your muscles.

This type of exercise is also beneficial in that it is low impact exercise and there is very little risk of injury. *Low impact* refers to exercise that puts little or low stress on your knees and ankles. Care should be taken to wear comfortable shoes so that this will remain as safe as possible. You will also benefit from some stretching exercises prior to your dancing activities.

If you feel awkward at first, realize that every one was a beginner at one point. Once you have practiced a few times, you will probably begin to experience a real aerobic workout and your coordination should improve. You should notice an improvement in your balance, posture, and your grace. Dancing will also help reduce your stress and anxiety level.

If you want to make this a special activity each week, join a class with some of your friends that struggle with weight problems. This type of exercise provides a good opportunity for recreation and meeting new people. Perhaps while you're losing the inches you can be gaining a friend.

34 NO MORE SHAME ON YOU

The term "shame on you" has a haunting tone to many people who feel condemned because of their lack of control in certain areas of their life. Many feel shame because of their weight. And the shame they feel makes the problem increase exponentially.

The Principle People who receive treatment for compulsive overeating are introduced to the concept of shame. Until people get in touch with the shame they feel, it will serve as the barrier to the road to recovery.

The primary shame most frequently identified in compulsive overeaters is a shame over a sense of perceived weakness with regard to self-control or a shame over their imperfection. Their overweight body becomes a constant reminder of their weakness and inferiority in being unable to reach an ideal body weight.

Idealization is a key factor here. People have ideals and goals that they use to set standards. Those with compulsive eating disorders do not perceive the ideal as a guideline, but rather as the goal. They look inwardly at their own lack of assertiveness as proof of inherent weakness. When individuals perceive their real self as nothing, loneliness and a fear of abandonment prevails. The basic human need to be connected or affiliated with others is severely threatened.

So, in an effort to show others that they are in control, strong, rational and logical, the person with a compulsive eating disorder will try to breach from their substandard self and mold into the image of what is idealized. They try to show others that they are not needy, angry, or unhappy. They believe that this near-perfect behavior will get them the love, approval, and acceptance for which they've always searched.

The Action Seek help through individual, group or in-patient therapy to overcome the shame you are feeling—whether your overeating problem is a result of sexual abuse, neglect or a problem of which you are not even aware. Find a group which deals with compulsive overeating and encourages writing assignments. Those involved are helped through a process of getting in touch with specific areas of shame and with their family systems to see how this affected their shame-based identity.

These sessions help people move toward freedom by making them aware of the shameful attitudes they have internalized regarding their inner selves and their bodies. And they can start people who hurt on a program that will do more than any "fad" diet. It will be the first step in an investment toward a permanent freedom from food.

35 HOW DRY I AM

"Oh no," you say. "Now they're going to ask me to stop drinking." Speaking from experience it can be done. With over 13 years of complete abstinence from alcohol between us we can assure you life goes on—and the weight comes off!

The Principle Perhaps you have been told that a glass of wine with a meal helps the digestion. That simply is not true. If anything, alcohol retards the digestion of food. It also creates a heavy burden on our liver and kidneys. Just as alcohol slows down your motor skills, it also slows your digestive system.

The Action Give up your consumption of wine and other alcoholic beverages. Alcohol contains calories that will add new pounds to your weight problem. And, if you already have an addiction to food, you are more likely to develop an addition to alcohol than are those people not involved in other addictions.

Alcohol, in addition to being a major source of weight gain, can have a negative effect on your emotional, physical, and spiritual health. It is a silent killer of relationships and lives in our world today. If you have a dependency upon alcohol and are reading this book to lose weight you should start by seeking treatment for your alcohol addiction today. A program like New Life Treatment

Centers will help you face both your addiction to food and alcohol. Call **1-800-227-LIFE** if you have **any** feelings that you might be addicted to alcohol, other drugs, or overeating.

36 MORNING GLORY

Your morning doesn't have to be a time of mourning. Here's a way to spice it up.

The Principle Breakfast does not have to be boring! There are ways to exchange certain ingredients in the foods you make with others that are lower in calories, fat, cholesterol, and sodium. You may be used to enjoying pastries and rolls with coffee in the morning hours. Even though the ideal weight-loss plan would probably exclude all sweets, you can actually still enjoy some of the sweet parts of your diet as long as you learn to eat them in moderation and always search for ways to reduce the calorie content. Chances are, you can give up sweets for a short time as part of a "fad" diet. We suggest that you learn a *lifelong* habit of rethinking your patterns and the way that you eat.

The Action An average bran muffin has approximately 175 to 200 calories. A low-fat yogurt has approximately 170 calories per serving. Here's a way to make reduced calorie cinnamon rolls that will each have approximately 141 calories.

Cinnamon Rolls

1 cup skim milk
3 tablespoons sugar
3 tablespoons margarine
  (divided)
1 package dry yeast
1/4 cup warm water (105° to
  115°)
1 egg, beaten
1/2 teaspoon salt

3 3/4 cups and 2 tablespoons
  bread flour
Vegetable cooking spray
1/4 cup plus 2 tablespoons
  firmly packed brown sugar
1 tablespoon skim milk
1/2 teaspoon vanilla extract
2 tablespoons ground cinnamon

Heat milk over medium-high heat in a heavy saucepan to 180° or until tiny bubbles form around edge (do not boil). Remove from heat.

Add sugar and one tablespoon margarine, stirring until margarine melts. Let cool until warm (105° to 115 °).

Dissolve yeast in warm water in a large bowl. Let stand for five minutes. Add milk mixture, egg, and salt. Stir well.

Gradually stir in 3 1/2 cups flour to make a soft dough. Turn out onto a lightly floured surface and knead until smooth and elastic (about eight minutes). Add flour, one tablespoon at a time, to keep dough from sticking to the surface.

Place the dough in a large bowl coated with cooking spray. Cover and let rise in a warm place that is free from drafts. Allow to rise until double in bulk.

Punch down dough. Turn out onto a lightly floured surface. Roll into a 20-by-8 inch rectangle. Brush two tablespoons melted margarine over the entire surface.

Sprinkle brown sugar and cinnamon evenly over dough.

Beginning at the longest side, roll dough up tightly, pinching the seam to seal. Do not seal the ends of the roll.

Cut the roll into 20 one-inch slices. Arrange slices in a pan coated with cooking spray. Cover and let rise in a warm place approximately thirty minutes.

Bake at 350° for 22 minutes. Combine powdered sugar, milk, and vanilla; stir well. Glaze mixture over rolls.

This recipe makes 20 rolls.

37 DEAR DIARY

Since the only person who can really control the way you eat is the one reading these words right now, help yourself maintain that accountability by tracking your foods and your personal progress in a daily diary.

The Principle If you are overweight, there are probably some things in your life that are out of control. Part of taking that control back is finding out how you got there in the first place and how your emotions are connected to your eating habits. Denial plays a major role in any unhealthy habit in which we are involved. Facing your denial with regard to overeating or unhealthy eating is the first step. Keeping a daily journal of what you eat and a daily diary of what you feel will help you overcome your denial and head you in the direction of wholeness and healing.

The Action Record daily what you are eating and what you are feeling in a journal. You can purchase a journal or simply make your own using a three-ring notebook, several tabs, and some lined paper. Label one tab "daily food journal" and label another "daily personal diary".

Daily Food Journal

On a daily basis record everything you eat. You will probably be surprised at just how much food you consume. And, the reality of seeing all you've eaten on paper may help you break down the denial and turn toward solutions to overcoming your weight problem. You might want to set up something for each day that looks like this:

Day	Date	Foods Eaten	Amount
		Breakfast:	
		Lunch:	
		Dinner:	
		Between Meals:	

Daily Personal Diary

At bedtime, write the date in your diary and describe your day. Write about your ups and downs, the difficult situations you faced or the moments of personal achievement. It may not be easy at first to be vulnerable and transparent—even with yourself.

But try your best to be as honest and realistic as you can.

Weekly Review

At the end of every week—review both of your diaries. (If weekends are the days when you eat the most, try doing your review on Friday night to give you extra willpower at the start of your toughest two days.) You will find out a great deal about yourself as you review the words you've written and the foods you've eaten.

Look in your diary for the days when you have more emotional lows, disappointments or rejections than usual. Then go to your food journal and see what you ate that day. If you find that you eat more snacks, desserts, and larger quantities of unhealthy food at meals on the rough days, you have made the first step in seeing that your extra weight may be a result of emotional hurts. You may be using food as a personal "reward" to yourself for facing such awful situations.

At the end of each week, take your food journal and use it to set up your plan for the following week. Delete the foods you know aren't good for you and replace them with lower-calorie foods. Use a calorie book to help you with this process.

Keep your journal and your diary with you wherever you go and continue tracking your eating habits. As you begin to trim back on your food you'll find it is helpful to write in your diary more than once a day. It is better to write about your feelings in your journal than it is to "stuff" the feelings inside by "stuffing" your stomach with more food. It is a process of finding out who the "real you" really is!

If the process of finding out the real you on your own scares you, call a professional or join a group to help you through the process.

38 HAMBURGER HELPER?

"But I don't feel like cooking a healthy meal tonight. I think I'll go for the old stand by at the local fast-food place. Ah! A hamburger, french fries, and a thick chocolate shake. What's a few more calories?"

The Principle We all seem to have our favorite place for the best burger in the world. A basic cheeseburger and order of french fries contains approximately 745 calories. So your goal in this chapter is to take your favorite foods, lower the calories and create a meal that you still will find satisfying and delicious.

Ground beef is loaded with fat and ingredients that add unnecessary calories. French fries are made from potatoes, a food that is naturally low in calories. Yet when deep fried, potatoes become high in fat content and loaded with calories. And what are french fries without a little salt which adds unwanted sodium to your system for water retention and catsup which contains sugar for even more calories? It all sounds delicious, but if you are like most people, after a meal like this your body can feel the effects.

The Action Americans spend thousands of dollars buying products that are reduced in calories, sodium, and cholesterol. Products with less, cost more. You have to pay more for mayonnaise with lower cholesterol, or for the crackers with lower sodium and the coffee without caffeine.

We recommend that you save money on these products and learn ways to substitute items high in fat and cholesterol with alternate foods that will be better for you.

Let's take the meal suggested at the beginning of this chapter and see how we can substitute some of the items.

The Hamburger

Mix together one pound of lean ground turkey, one egg, one chopped onion, two tablespoons of a no-salt seasoning and one tablespoon of garlic powder. Mold these ingredients together to make turkey patties. You can either barbecue them or fry them in a pan sprayed with a non-oil spray. If you must eat your turkey with a bun, select one that is high in fiber and low in calories. Instead of catsup, use low-calorie 1,000 island dressing or salsa. Garnish your burger with lettuce and tomato.

The Fries

Instead of french fries, make oven-baked fries. Slice a peeled potato into french fries or steak fries. Preheat the oven to 450 degrees. Lightly grease a cooking tin or glass pan with diet margarine. Lay your potatoes side by side without piling them on top of one another. Sprinkle garlic powder and no-salt seasoning over the potatoes. Bake for 30 to 40 minutes turning them over once or twice until browned. These potatoes will taste great and will be much healthier for you than if they were fried. For a special treat, dip the fries in low-calorie ranch dressing instead of catsup, or sprinkle on a small portion of a butter substitute or Parmesan cheese.

Replace the milk shake with herbal iced tea and lemon.

Eating more healthy meals may be an adjustment at first. But the more you learn to substitute salts with other spices, beef with leaner options and sodas with mineral waters, the more weight you will lose and the better you will feel about your health.

39 "NUR"TRI-TION

A woman once had a condition
She ate lots but not for nutrition
To help her heart mend
She called to a friend
Who brought her a new found fruition

The Principle Because overweight people often use food to nurture themselves, they must stop these unhealthy patterns and learn healthy new ways to nurture themselves.

The Action As part of your recovery process as an overeater, you must take an honest look at your relationship with food. See if it is merely a means of nutritional survival or if it has become something more.

One of the toughest parts of being human is that we sometimes face the break ups of relationships or friendships. This process usually happens in stages. In most cases, we begin by struggling with an uneasiness knowing that something is wrong in a friendship. Then we search within to try and discover why we are not feeling quite right about ourselves or our relationship with the other person. Next, we make a decision to confront the other person and the problem between us and break off the relationship. We then grieve the loss and allow time to heal the pain.

If you feel like you are in a relationship with food rather than merely seeing it as a means of nutrition then follow these same stages to break up with your friend named Food. The very realization of facing the truth that you must make that move can begin the deep work of healing within your heart and soul. Facing the real truth and breaking through the denial in our lives is the spark that can ignite the flame of hope toward recovery. If you have been searching for the truth to your problem, perhaps you're finding it at this very moment.

There is great comfort in truth. Many people have a tendency to beat themselves up for overeating, thinking that they are all bad and have no good within them. But, in reality, they have been hurt or still hurt—and lacking trust in others they find safety only in their best friend that won't hurt them—food. This is where the dysfunction sets in. Because food will and does hurt the overeater. And it will never be a good friend. Food is not meant for relationships. It is a source of nutrition. That's it. Only people can provide healthy relationships.

Here are a few tips to develop new and healthy relationships:

- Survey your relationship with food and develop a healthy perspective on this nutritional substance.
- Inventory your relationships with those around you. Think about the people you know from work, home, school, church, and organizations in which you are involved. Find ways to strengthen healthy relationships and repair

those that have been damaged. Consider phasing out friendships that have been destructive.

- Look at your own skills for relating to people. Consider counseling to make the changes you need to relate better.
- Find new healthy relationships that will be supportive, accepting, and loving. Nurture yourself in the same way.
- Give yourself time and be patient. Going from unhealthy relationships to healthy ones is a process. Give yourself that chance by taking one day at a time.

40 CHECK THE THER-MOSTAT

You've tried everything including near starvation to lose weight, yet the scale still says that same old thing—maybe even more. Now what do you do?

The Principle Failure to lose weight despite all efforts can sometimes be traced to an underactive thyroid gland, a kind of thermostat in the body that alters our energy. People who struggle with obesity often undergo routine tests for thyroid functions. But there are also many who have self-diagnosed themselves with this problem to deny the fact that they overeat each and every day.

The Action When you combine excessive calorie intake and an underactive thyroid you can have other problems such as constipation and fatigue in addition to obesity. If you suspect that you may have this problem, consult a doctor and ask him or her to run thyroid tests. Treatment for an underactive thyroid can enable you to escape from starvation diets and still lose weight.

Low carbohydrate diets often work well for people that don't respond to ordinary reducing diets. Six small meals a day will be easier for you to digest and will usually make weight maintenance or weight loss easier. Here is an example of a one-day low carbohydrate diet.

Breakfast

One serving of fresh fruit
One egg or egg substitute
A half-slice of thin whole wheat toast

Snack

One glass of skimmed milk
One cup of coffee or tea (optional)
(No sugar, cream, or regular milk)

Lunch

One helping of lean meat, fish, or fowl
One serving of vegetables
One small salad

Snack

One serving of fruit
One cup of herbal tea

Dinner

One cup of soup
One helping of lean meat, fish, or fowl
Two vegetables

Snack

Unsweetened fruit cocktail
One cup of tea

In order to better plan a low carbohydrate diet, purchase a carbohydrate guide and plan your six smaller meals each day. If you have tried all sorts of diets with little or no results, it is time to contact your physician for thyroid and other tests.

41 BEHAVIOR MODIFI- CATION

It's the little things that count.

The Principle As you continue to develop a plan for losing weight, it is important that you change some of your behaviors and patterns. There are simple things you can do to avoid over-eating, facing temptations, and diverting from your plan.

The Action Here are some things you can do to stay on course and modify your eating behaviors:

- During meal times focus your attention upon the food you are eating and nothing else. Enjoy the taste and texture of your food. Avoid watching television, talking on the phone, or reading. Since you should only eat three times a day, make the best of these times.
- Make the area where you eat most of your meals a special place, whether it is in your dining room or kitchen nook. Add comfort to this place by displaying fresh flowers, playing soft music and using the best silverware and dishes. Reserve this special place only for mealtimes so that you will not eat at home in

between meals. Since it will be a place where you are comfortable, let it help you feel better about the progress you are making.

- Eat from a smaller plate than you are used to. The larger the plate you use, the more you are likely to put on it.
- If you don't eat all of your food, either discard it or freeze it. Unfrozen leftovers are too tempting to eat as a snack in the evening or in between meals.
- Avoid the routes that cause you to stumble and overeat. If the normal road you take home from work or school is lined with ice cream shops or fast-food restaurants, begin taking an alternate route that is "safer" for you.
- When going to the market, do not put foods that are tempting to you in the shopping cart. Better yet, shop at a health food store so that there are not as many temptations.

So that you can specifically work on some of the little things that cause you to slip from your course, we've provided space to list those things that make you overeat or eat the wrong foods. Work on ways to break the chains of old habits and learn new behaviors!

Old habit: _____
New behavior to avoid this old habit: _____
_____
Old habit: _____

New behavior to avoid this old habit: _____

_____

Old habit: _____
New behavior to avoid this old habit: _____

_____

42 FRUIT BEFORE NOON

If you follow this idea carefully, you may find yourself losing unwanted weight in the very first week!

The Principle When eaten on an empty stomach, fresh fruit accelerates weight loss. Your body and digestive tract are set up on cycles to digest foods and to eliminate them from your system. Some people think that fruit and fruit juices are fattening. When fruit is altered by heat or incorrectly consumed with or immediately following certain other foods, it can have negative effects on your weight.

Calories are enemies only if they are consumed in foods highly processed or improperly combined. Quality calories such as those found in high-water-content foods in most cases will not add more weight. Instead, they will give you more energy to do away with extra weight.

The Action In this method of losing weight you will not focus so much on counting calories as you will on combining your foods in a manner that results in low-energy digestion and in a "fuel efficient" manner. This is tied closely to the effective functioning of your body cycles. The "elimination" cycle takes place approximately from 4:00 a.m. until noon.

By eating nothing but fruit during these hours your body will try to eliminate the calories. Eating other types of foods during this cycle can add unwanted pounds rather than eliminate them. This is partially due to the fact that fruit demands the least amount of energy for digestion.

The intestines are the place where all nutrients are absorbed. Since fruit finds its way into the intestines within minutes instead of hours, nutrients are immediately absorbed and utilized by your body. You will probably find that when you eat nothing but fruit before noon, your day will be filled with more energy.

And, even if you don't stay on a well-planned food program all day eating only *fresh* fruit and drinking only *fresh* fruit juices before noon will help you reduce your weight. If you must have coffee on this plan you will have to wait until after noon to drink it.

43 DINNER SALAD

If you are used to making dinner the big meal of the day, the dinner may be making you the "big" deal of today.

The Principle   Toward the end of the day we have the tendency to eat our heaviest meal and then relax from a busy day. Because the evening meal is followed within hours of the time of day we lay down for a good night's sleep, it is the absolute worst time to absorb a high number of calories. The evening meal should be our lightest meal. And, reducing the number of calories you eat in the evening should be a big step in your weight-loss plan.

The Action   Your evening meal should be easy to digest and low in calories. We recommend eating a salad. As suggested in the "Trip to the Salad Bar" chapter, you should purchase or mix your own low-calorie dressings for these meals. And, as a general rule, do not include high-calorie toppings such as cheeses and nuts.

You may think that a salad every night for dinner will be boring. But you can be very creative with this meal. Here are some suggestions to get you started.

Vegetable Garden Salad

Combine lettuce, carrots, celery, tomatoes, cucumbers, onions, sprouts, and one hard-boiled egg (for protein) into a bowl. Sprinkle on some garlic powder and lemon pepper for flavor. Add a small portion of your favorite low-calorie dressing.

Charbroiled Chicken Salad

Add to an assortment of pea pods, water chestnuts, sprouts, and tomatoes a charbroiled chicken breast chopped up into tasty bite-sized pieces. Place ingredients over a bed of lettuce. Mix in your favorite spices and dressing.

Tuna Salad

Start with a can of water-packed, low salt tuna fish. Toss the tuna with lettuce, tomatoes, celery, onions, cucumbers, and black olives. For variety, stuff these ingredients inside a large tomato before serving.

Shrimp Salad

Toss lettuce, tomato, cucumbers, onions, celery, sprouts, and some fresh shrimp. Mix together with your favorite spices and low-calorie dressing.

Fresh Vegetable Salad

Chop up fresh broccoli, carrots, cauliflower, tomatoes, and a small portion of low-fat cheese. Add your spices and dressing.

Spinach Salad

Mix together fresh spinach leaves with regular or romaine lettuce. Add orange slices, spices, and the whites of one hard-boiled egg (yokes contain the fat and unwanted calories—whites contain the protein and low-fat calories). Top your salad lightly with a low-calorie Italian dressing or vinegar and oil.

Fruit Salad

Slice strawberries, orange sections, pineapple, honeydew melons, apples, and raisins. Place fruit on a bed of lettuce and top with your favorite low-fat yogurt.

Now you have a variety of ways to serve salads for your evening meal. We've provided seven— enough for a different salad every day of the week. List below on separate recipe cards three of your own suggestions for additional salad ideas.

44 TWO-WAY CONVER-SATION

*For it is God who works in you both to
will and to do for His good pleasure.*
Philippians 2:13

The Principle   Once we have admitted to ourselves that we are powerless when it comes to
food, we need to acknowledge a power which is
greater than ourselves. While support groups and
the buddy system will give us encouragement that
we need to lose weight, it is only through God our
Creator that the real changes within us can take
place. And, just as time together is the only way we
can really get to know a fellow human being, time
with God is the only way to know Him.

The Action   Meditate upon the scriptures that
God has given to us. Search for those that are particularly helpful to your pain and situation. As you
read each scripture, make notes reflecting your
prayers back to God. You may even want to add a
section to the journal and diary we presented in an
earlier chapter. For example one of our favorite
scriptures from the book of Matthew is:

> Come to Me, all you who labor and are heavy laden,
> and I will give you rest. Take My yoke upon you and
> learn from Me, for I am gentle and lowly in heart,

> and you will find rest for your souls. For My yoke is
> easy and My burden is light. Matthew 11:28–30

And your response might be:

> God, Your word brings me comfort but I need to
> truly experience freedom from this burden I feel. I
> need the rest that You describe in this passage. I
> have carried this burden so long that I need Your
> help in releasing the pain. I am asking that You min-
> ister to me because You created me and are the only
> who knows exactly where I am in my struggle.

By using this method you will be having a two-
way conversation with your Creator—listening to
His word and then responding with your reply. If
you find intimate relationships difficult, you may
have trouble asking God to intimately come in to
your life. But allowing God to take your burden is
the key to your freedom from it.

Here are some further scriptures which you
might find comforting.

> For I am persuaded that neither death nor life, nor
> angels nor principalities nor things present nor
> things to come, nor height nor depth, nor any other
> created thing, shall be able to separate us from the
> love of God which is in Christ Jesus our Lord. Ro-
> mans 8:38–39

> Fear not, for I am with you; be not dismayed, for I
> am your God. I will strengthen you, yes, I will help
> you, I will uphold you with My righteous right hand.
> Isaiah 41:10

For God so loved the world that He gave His only begotten Son, that whoever believes in Him should not perish but have everlasting life. For God did not send His Son into the world to condemn the world, but that the world through Him might be saved. John 3:16–17

Trust in the Lord with all your heart, and lean not on your own understanding; in all your ways acknowledge Him, and He shall direct your paths. Proverbs 3:5–6

Teach me to do Your will, for You are my God; Your Spirit is good. Lead me in the land of uprightness. Psalm 143:10

Commit your works to the Lord, and your thoughts will be established. Proverbs 16:3

Most assuredly, I say to you, he who believes in Me, the works that I do he will do also; and greater works than these he will do, because I go to My Father. And whatever you ask in My name, that I will do, that the Father may be glorified in the Son. John 14:12–13

For I know the thoughts that I think toward you, says the Lord, thoughts of peace and not of evil, to give you a future and a hope. Then you will call upon Me and go and pray to Me, and I will listen to you. And you will seek Me and find Me, when you search for Me with all your heart. I will be found by you, says the Lord, . . . Jeremiah 29:11–14a

45 THE PLATEAU

Sometime during your weight loss plan, after several consistent weeks of losing a few pounds, you may hit a period where your efforts seem to have no results. Do not lose heart. Some call it "the plateau". You may feel like you've hit a wall.

The Principle Often, after about two months of eating properly and exercising regularly, you step on the scale and see little or no more improvement. Do *not* interpret this as a personal failure or as a sign of your lacking willpower and dedication. It is a sign of something completely natural happening within your system that is a very common occurrence with people trying to lose weight.

The Action In Chapter Fourteen entitled "A Mighty Metabolism" we explained that your body will often slow down due to the fact that you have been taking in fewer calories. As part of that chapter, we suggested that you continue with a regular exercise plan to help step up your metabolism.

The natural reaction with regard to your food consumption is to eat less in hopes of getting the scale to continue dropping. Some people even border on starving themselves. If you try these actions, chances are you will feel so uncomfortable and irritable that you'll quit all the good habits that have been formed out of frustration. And chances are you will gain the weight back as quickly as you lost it.

Instead of taking drastic measures, the best thing to do is continue with the plan you've been on for the past few weeks or months. Your body should readjust and the weight again should continue to come off. There isn't much you can do during one of these periods except continue with your healthy eating and regular exercise and wait it out.

To deal with your emotional state of mind, avoid feeling guilty or discouraged that things have slowed down. Instead, pat yourself on the back for all the great progress you've made thus far. Even if you hit "the wall" as early as the second week of your new plan, focus inwardly on the process you've started rather than outwardly on the actual goal. If you have been eating properly and exercising even for a short time, you can affirm yourself by recognizing the new energy you feel and the increase in your self-esteem that has been generated through the few pounds you've already lost.

One last bit of advice during this time. Put the scale away for a couple of weeks while you maintain your program. During times like this it can be your worst friend. Focus your attention on the victories you are accomplishing.

46 WATER RATIONING

Remember when your mother used to tell you to drink lots of water? Well, she was right.

The Principle Since all of our bodies are different, some people are more inclined to retain water in their systems than are others. The bloated feeling that sometimes accompanies water retention can be a discouraging frustration to people who are dieting. Often water retention causes people to give up their diets or turn to prescription diuretics. These medications can become addicting and most drain your body of essential vitamins and minerals.

The Action During the times when we feel bloated, the normal tendency is to stop drinking water and refrain from eating high-water-content foods. In fact, this is the very time when we should increase our water intake. Many people who do not have weight problems claim it is partially due to the fact that daily they drink a great deal of water.

It is a well-known fact that large amounts of water consumed on a daily basis will flush out unwanted poisons and toxins from our bodies. That is one reason that you are to rest in bed and "drink plenty of fluids" when you are ill. Water also helps to flush out waste materials in our intestines.

Women will usually experience temporary water-weight gain once a month for a week to ten days. We recommend the use of **natural** diuretics at this time or any time you feel that you're experiencing water retention. Here are some ideas that might work for you.

Iced Tea

Drinking iced tea with lemon will increase your water intake and flush more fluids from your system.

Hot Water

Hot water with lemon juice is very effective for reducing water retention in some people. Add flavor to your cup of hot water with concentrated pure lemon juice.

Apples

Still another idea for dealing with water retention is to consume peeled large Granny Smith or large pippin apples or any other large apples.

Consult your physician if your water retention problem is severe, prolonged, or causing you a great deal of frustration.

47 WEIGHT AWHILE

In addition to your aerobic exercise, get involved in some light but regular weight training to further tone your muscles.

The Principle Although all exercise involves a degree of stress, weight training applies this stress to your muscles in a controlled manner. Most forms of exercise do not focus on a specific muscle group in your body, but rather help improve your overall fitness. Proper weight training allows you to focus on a specific part of your body that you would like to tone. For example, you can work specifically on your arms and shoulders through weight exercises that build your upper body.

The Action Since weight training does not produce any significant improvement to your cardiovascular system, it is important that you are also involved in one of the aerobic exercises described in this book. These two, working hand in hand, will help you lose weight and then tone the specific parts of your body that you want to improve. For example, you may combine an hour of speed walking with some weight training focusing on your upper thighs. Of course, you must stick to your new food habits in addition to these two forms of fitness training.

Be sure to see a physician first and have a trained expert help you set up a weight program that is appropriate for your needs and level of strength. You may want to try a few different exercises to avoid boredom. And as you reach various plateaus, your trainer can change your program to promote further progress.

Your workout will vary according to such factors as:

- The frequency of your workouts
- Your current energy level
- The amount of rest you have been getting
- The amount of weight you are lifting
- The number of repetitions you are making
- The duration of your rest periods
- Your diet

Check with your local health club instructor to see what workout program he or she recommends for your body.

48 I'LL TAKE THE LOW ROAD

Each time you journey toward another meal, there are decisions to make. You can select the road filled with "high" fat foods or take the road "low" in fat and cholesterol.

The Principle   Certain foods that we eat every day contain significant levels of fat and cholesterol. Not only do foods high in fat and cholesterol contribute to our weight gain, but they can cause serious health problems even to the person who appears to have very little excess weight.

The Action   Instead of eating foods high in fat and cholesterol, begin substituting the items you normally eat with alternate foods. The chart below offers some of those substitutions. For further weight loss, you can learn to live without some of the substitute items altogether.

High-Fat Item	Low-Fat Substitute
Apple pie	Sugarless pippin applesauce with granola sprinkled on top
Bacon, sausage	Lean turkey sausage, lean turkey bacon
Bologna	Chicken or turkey bologna

Butter, margarine	Apple butter, fruit spreads, and jams with no added sugar
Cheese and crackers	Rice cakes topped with apple butter
Cream, Half-and-Half	Nonfat milk, 2% milk, powdered milk
Donuts and sweet rolls	High-fiber, low-sugar bran or oat-bran muffins
Eggs	Egg whites only (yokes contain high fat)
Fried fish	Baked or broiled fish topped with lemon
Frosted cereals	Shredded Wheat or rice or bran cereals
Hamburgers	95 percent lean turkey burgers
Ice cream	Nonfat, unsweetened frozen yogurt
Macaroni and cheese	Pasta sprinkled with Parmesan cheese; butter substitute; no-salt seasoning
Mashed potatoes and gravy	Baked potato topped with low-calorie low-fat ranch dressing and chives
Mayonnaise, sour cream	Nonfat yogurt mixed with a small amount of nonfat buttermilk; mustard

49 ROAST BOAST

When you think of roasting, one of two things probably come to mind—the Thanksgiving turkey or the comedy of Don Rickles. Here are a few more ideas to add to your roasting repertoire.

The Principle If you are like many Americans, the only time you had a roasted dinner was during the holidays when turkey was served or occasionally a Sunday pot roast. Memories of these meals are probably flavored with fondness, yet it probably seems that the preparation of such food took hours and hours. But this does not necessarily have to be the case.

The truth is, that at temperatures of 450° to 500°, you can cook fish, veal, whole chickens, peppers, mushrooms, or mixed vegetables in less time than it takes to stir-fry. And, even though there is intense heat involved, when your time is limited roasting still imparts intense flavor in the food.

One of the biggest benefits of roasting is that it draws out the fats in chicken, duck, or turkey. But care must be taken when roasting at high temperatures to ensure that the hot grease does not splatter against the walls of the roasting pan. A thick layer of kosher salt in the roasting pan will catch the drippings and avoid the problem of smoke in your kitchen. The salt will absorb the grease you might normally use for gravy. But since gravy contains a great deal of fat, you won't want these drippings for any reason.

The Action   Try roasting some of your favorite foods that you've never prepared this way before. Vegetables are more tasty when roasted. Combine your favorite spices and a light glaze of olive, peanut, or sesame seed oil and roast them until they are as soft as you like them.

Here is a guide to show you the temperature to roast some specific foods you might enjoy.

Roast at 500°

- Chickens, whole
- Grouper
- Mako shark
- Monk fish filets
- Salmon filets
- Scallops
- Swordfish
- Tuna

Roast at 450°

- Asparagus
- Eggplant
- Green beans
- Lamb chops
- Leeks
- Mushrooms
- Peppers
- Potatoes
- Shallots
- Veal chops
- Zucchini

50 IT'S CLEAR AS WATER

Perhaps you think that your bad back or weak ankles has provided you with an "out" when it comes to exercise such as jogging. That isn't the case. Swimming provides you a way to change your "out" by jumping "in" a pool.

The Principle   Swimming is an excellent aerobic exercise that, when done consistently, will help you get in great shape. It will help you strengthen your heart and lungs without the high impact on your muscles, tendons, and bones that accompanies such sports as jogging or a vigorous game of basketball. Swimming will help develop your arms, chest, shoulders, and legs to give you a well-balanced work-out and a better proportioned body.

The Action   Perhaps you already are on a walking or jogging program. Swimming can be a great addition to the routine of anyone, whether they currently work out or not. If you are not an experienced swimmer, you may want to spend some time with an instructor who will teach you the strokes, breathing techniques, and work-out programs to best help your progress.

If you do not have a pool available, check with your local YMCA, community center or health club to see if they have or know of a pool for public use in your area. As we've suggested throughout this book, consider finding a friend to swim laps with you. This will help you stay accountable and will further your fellowship time with this new or existing friend.

Begin your new work-out by swimming a few laps each day. Then as your endurance increases, build on the number of laps you swim each day. Here are some suggestions for your swimming program.

Water Stretching.

Prior to each swimming experience, do stretching exercises before and after you get in the water. Once in, hold yourself up at the side of the pool to stretch the muscles. This will help you relax as you swim and lessen the chances for cramps.

Water Ballet.

Some swimming clubs or health spas offer water ballet classes for those who want fun exercise while they swim. Find a friend and join a class together. In between classes, develop your own routines.

Ocean Swimming.

If you are fortunate to live near the ocean, try swimming parallel to the shore just beyond the swells. Of course, you should be an experienced swimmer and know the cautions of riptides and dangerous currents before attempting this kind of swimming.

Use a Snorkel and Mask.

Whether you are swimming in the ocean or in a pool, you might want to use a mask and snorkel. In the ocean, it will allow you to view the sea life below. In the pool it can help you if you have trouble with your neck or difficulty swimming without running out of breath. Before long people around you will probably be using their masks and snorkels along side of you.

Tread Water.

Another good aerobic exercise is treading water. Set a goal to tread water in a certain spot for a length of time. Alternate every few minutes between the following:

- Treading water with your arms and legs
- Treading water with just your legs—arms at your side
- Treading water with just your arms—legs at rest in the water

You may want to purchase an inexpensive waterproof watch or work out where there is a poolside clock so that you can do each of these for several minutes apiece. Compete with others to see who can tread water the longest.

Songs to Swim by.

If you enjoy music, there are products on the market, such as a waterproof radio, that will allow you to listen to music while you tread water. Or, if you are not disturbing others, bring a portable radio with you to the pool and water dance while you tread.

As you can see, there's more than one way to "swim a lap."

51 HELP

The weakest link is often the one which is hollow—it appears strong on the outside but is empty on the inside. The void can only be altered after the hollowness is discovered and the empty spaces begin to be filled.

The Principle   Part of the challenge presented here has been for you to come face-to-face with your behaviors and attitudes, not your eating patterns alone. Thousands of women and men are not going to find the answer in simple diets because they deal with a form of *bulimia* and are not even aware of it.

Bulimia is seen by the public as a behavior wherein the person binges on food and then either purges it or rids of it through the use of laxatives. But a bulimic can also be one who eats and then immediately goes to sleep. Or one who eats and tries to rid themselves of the food by overexercising. Some bulimics eat a lot of food and then starve themselves by missing the next few meals to make up for the excess food. It presents an overwhelming fear of being overweight—sometimes to the point of panic.

The Action   If you have any suspicion that you are fighting bulimia it is important that you get the help you need to win the battle. Suppose after months of dieting and exercise, with no results, you found out that you had a thyroid problem.

And, once treated you found that the special diet and exercise began working for you to the point that you reached total recovery.

Bulimia presents a similar situation in that the problem is *not* food. Bulimia is the result of deep-seeded issues which you may not even be in touch with. A bulimic person is *not* crazy. Rather, he or she needs specialized care in working through the issues of life to reduce their weight once and for all.

If you, or someone you know, has any of the behaviors or symptoms listed above, specialized treatment is needed for recovery. It can be the key to freedom for the rest of your or this person's life. Once you are out of treatment, you can use the 52 ways presented in this book to help maintain a plan for healthy exercise and diet.

> Being in recovery myself from bulimia I talk to women, men, children and their loved ones who are struggling with these issues in their own lives. If you have questions regarding your own possible eating disorder or have concerns for someone you love, please call me for a confidential conversation. I can be reached at **1-800-227-LIFE**.
>
> Mary E. Ehemann

52 WHAT DO YOU KNOW?

We hope the ideas we have shown
Include some new things you'll
  condone
Because you've got more
We'll give you the chore
Of writing a few of your own

The Principle It is our hope that many of the fifty-one ideas already presented will help you lose the weight that you want to lose. We've presented a lot of different ideas, in a wide variety of formats. But as you've read these pages, perhaps you've thought of some ideas that have worked for you in the past with regard to weight loss. In this chapter, we encourage you to record those ideas so that all of your weight loss plans—the ones we've presented and the ones you've developed are listed in one convenient place.

The Action In the spaces that follow, list some of the ways you have successfully lost weight in the past. If you have a method of losing weight you would like to share with us, please mail it to the address listed on the following page. We both sincerely hope that you have found these ideas encouraging to your weight loss goals and wish you all the best in developing a healthier you!

My Own Weight Loss Ideas

1. _____

_____

_____

2. _____

_____

_____

3. _____

_____

_____

4. _____

_____

_____

5. _____

_____

_____

Send your own weight loss ideas to:

Ways to Lose Weight
c/o Carl Dreizler
P. O. Box 4788
Laguna Beach, CA 92652